How To Manage REM Sleep Behavior Disorder

Practical Strategies for Thriving with Rapid Eye Movement RBD and Supporting Loved Ones

Denise R. Doty

Table of Content

Introduction

"Understanding and controlling Rapid Eye Movement (REM) Sleep Behavior Disorder (RBD) is critical to leading a full and productive life. This book is intended to walk you through every step of RBD, from detecting symptoms to establishing a supportive atmosphere for yourself and others around you. Whether you are recently diagnosed, supporting a loved one, or simply looking for information, this comprehensive resource strives to give clarity, emotional support, and practical assistance."

Imagine resting in bed, drifting off into a deep slumber, only to awaken to vivid and frequently violent nightmares. You kick, punch, and scream, waking up disoriented and maybe hurt. This is the reality for those with Rapid Eye Movement Sleep Behavior Disorder (RBD). RBD, which was discovered in the early 1980s, is still a relatively unknown yet profoundly significant disorder. Our understanding of RBD has advanced greatly over the last few decades, due in large part to pioneering researchers and courageous individuals who have shared their experiences.

RBD occurs when the brain's normal regulation of muscle activity during REM sleep fails. People with RBD physically act out their dreams rather than laying still during them. These acts might range from modest movements to risky habits that endanger both the sleeper and their bed mate. Understanding RBD entails delving into the science of sleep, the disorder's symptoms, and the larger consequences for health and well being.

The discovery of RBD was a watershed moment in the field of sleep medicine. It revealed the complex interplay between our cerebral functioning and sleep. Researchers discovered that RBD is frequently an early warning sign of neurodegenerative disorders including Parkinson's and Lewy body dementia. This link has created new opportunities for early detection and intervention, bringing hope for better management and treatment of many illnesses.

We understand that RBD may be frightening and isolating. Many persons with RBD feel misunderstood or unable to obtain appropriate therapies. This book aims to close the gap by providing clear, evidence based information and practical suggestions. We will go over everything from the fundamentals of sleep and REM cycles to the specifics of living with RBD on a daily basis.

Who this is book for

This book is for anybody who wants to better understand and handle RBDs. This book is for anybody who has been diagnosed with RBD, suspects they may have it, or is a caregiver or family member of someone suffering from the illness. We want to give practical, actionable information that will help you negotiate the obstacles of RBD and enhance your quality of life.

Individuals with RBD will discover extensive descriptions of the illness, methods for managing symptoms, and information on how to seek medical attention. Our objective is to provide you with information and methods to help you regulate your illness and live a satisfying life.

For caregivers and family members, understanding RBD is critical for delivering appropriate care. This book will teach you how to spot symptoms, create a secure atmosphere, and effectively communicate with a loved one. We also discuss the emotional and psychological effects of caregiving and provide advice on how to preserve your own well being.

For healthcare professionals: If you are a doctor, therapist, or sleep expert, this book provides a thorough explanation of RBD, including the most recent studies and treatments. Our goal is to assist you diagnose and treat this difficult condition so that you can deliver the best treatment possible to your patients.

This book is an excellent resource for academics and students researching sleep medicine, neurology, and psychology. We present an in depth look at the mechanics of RBD, its links to neurodegenerative illnesses, and existing knowledge gaps that future research might fill.

Chapter 1

What is REM Sleep Behavior Disorder

To comprehend REM Sleep Behavior Disorder (RBD), you must first understand the fundamentals of sleep itself. Sleep is not a single condition, but rather a complicated process that goes through several stages. The phases include light sleep, deep sleep, and Rapid Eye Movement (REM) sleep. REM sleep is very significant because it is when most of our dreams occur.

The brain is extremely active during REM sleep, almost as if you are awake, yet the body is usually paralyzed for a short period of time. This paralysis, known as REM atonia, keeps you from acting on your fantasies. It's the brain's method of protecting you while you sleep. REM sleep is essential for cognitive processes including memory consolidation, learning, and emotional control.

However, for those with RBD, this paralysis does not develop as expected. Instead, the muscles stay engaged, and the individual can physically play out their fantasies. This may entail talking, shouting, striking, kicking, and even getting out of bed and moving about. These activities can be shocking and hazardous, resulting in injury to both the person with RBD and their bed partner.

Definition and characteristics of RBD.

REM Sleep Behavior Disorder is characterized by the absence or incompleteness of the typical paralysis that occurs during REM sleep, allowing the individual to move and act out their dreams. RBD is classified as a parasomnia, which is a sleep condition characterized by aberrant movements, actions, emotions, perceptions, or dreams.

The features of RBD are fairly unique.

1. Dream Enactment: People with RBD frequently act out vivid and dramatic dreams. These nightmares might

be violent, prompting behaviors like kicking, hitting, or running.

2. Injury danger: Because the motions are quick and strong, there is a high danger of injury. This involves slipping out of bed, striking adjacent objects, or inadvertently injuring a bedmate.

3. Sleep Disruption: Physical exercise may trigger frequent awakenings, resulting in poor sleep quality and increased daytime drowsiness.

4. People with RBD may talk, yell, or scream while sleeping. These vocalizations are frequently in reaction to the dream material.

5. RBD bouts might occur sometimes or numerous times per night. The issue might develop and worsen over time.

The Discovery of RBD from the Historical Perspective

The identification of RBD is a relatively new finding in sleep medicine. It was initially described in the 1980s by a group of researchers at a sleep disorders facility.

Previously, RBD related behaviors were frequently misinterpreted or misdiagnosed.

The discovery occurred when a group of patients displayed odd and aggressive actions while sleeping. These actions were originally surprising since they did not follow the conventional patterns of established sleep disorders like sleepwalking or night terrors. Researchers determined that the activities originated during REM sleep, a period when the body is ordinarily immobilized.

One of the first published examples concerned a retired person who began having intense and violent nightmares in which he physically acted out. On one occasion, he attacked a dresser as if he were playing football. This instance was significant because it revealed a previously unknown syndrome, necessitating a new understanding of REM sleep and its mechanics.

The study not only established RBD as a unique condition but also demonstrated its potential as an early warning sign of neurodegenerative disorders including

Parkinson's and Lewy body dementia. This link has important implications for early detection and management, providing a window of opportunity to address these disorders before more severe symptoms appear.

The discovery and study of RBD has opened up new avenues in sleep research and neurology. Understanding the fundamental causes of RBD has resulted in more effective diagnostic tools and treatment alternatives, bringing relief and safety to people affected.

Chapter 2

Recognizing Symptoms of RBD

Recognizing the signs of REM Sleep Behavior Disorder (RBD) is critical for timely diagnosis and treatment. RBD symptoms range from moderate to severe, with strength and frequency changing by individual. Understanding these symptoms can assist in recognizing the disease and obtaining proper medical treatment.

1. Dream Enactment Behavior: The most distinguishing feature of RBD is the physical enactment of dreams. This includes talking, shouting, gesturing, striking, kicking, and even jumping out of bed. These behaviors mirror the dream's content, which is frequently vivid and dramatic.

2. Vocalizations: People with RBD may produce a variety of noises while sleeping. This may involve

chatting, yelling, screaming, or even laughing. These vocalizations are typically tied to what is happening in the dream and can be rather loud, upsetting both the individual and their bed companion.

3. Individuals with RBD frequently wake up because of their physical activity and vocalizations. They may wake up several times every night, resulting in poor sleep quality and increased daytime drowsiness.

4. Injuries: One of the most dangerous features of RBD is the possibility of injury. Both the individual with RBD and their bedmate may be injured during these episodes. Bruises, scrapes, and even fractures are common injuries caused by falls or furniture accidents.

5. dread and worry: The vivid and frequently violent character of the nightmares can cause dread and worry. People with RBD may wake up feeling upset or scared, and their bed companions may be nervous about sleeping next to someone with unexpected movements.

6. Memory of Dreams: Unlike some other sleep disorders, people with RBD frequently recall their dreams in full. This recall is attributable to the vividness of the dreams and the partial awakenings that occur throughout episodes.

Real Life Experiences

Hearing about real life stories will help you better grasp how RBD appears and impacts people's lives. Here are a few case examples that demonstrate the diversity of experiences persons with RBD may have:

1. The Fighter: A retired office worker began having vivid dreams about violent conflicts. In one dream, he defended himself against an assailant. His wife awoke to see him flinging fists into the air, nearly missing her face. On another occasion, he kicked the nightstand, causing a damaged toe. These bouts occurred many times every month, leaving him fatigued and anxious to retire to bed.

2. The Runner: A lady in her sixties began experiencing nightmares about fleeing from danger. She would frequently rush out of bed, occasionally bashing against walls or furniture. One night, she collided with a dresser, sustaining a serious cut on her forehead. These occurrences caused substantial sleep disruption and required many clinic appointments for injuries.

3. Another gentleman wants to safeguard his family from invaders. While still unconscious, he would cry warnings and violently defend himself against imagined attacks. His loud ranting and aggressive actions worried his wife, who was fearful of being accidentally wounded during these outbursts. Following many nights of interrupted sleep and increased worry, the couple sought medical attention.

Differentiating RBD from Other Sleep Disorders.

RBD has several parallels with other sleep disorders, making it difficult to diagnose without expert guidance.

However, there are certain major distinctions that distinguish RBD:

1. Sleepwalking and RBD are both physical movements that occur during sleep, but during distinct periods of the sleep cycle. Sleepwalking occurs during non REM sleep and usually includes more instinctive, less sophisticated movements such as walking or moving around the house. RBD, on the other hand, occurs during REM sleep and consists of more intricate and frequently violent dream related behaviors.

2. Night Terrors: These are unexpected awakenings accompanied by great panic, screaming, and thrashing. They often occur during non REM sleep, particularly in the first portion of the night. People who have night terrors are typically not fully aware and may not recall the incident in the morning. RBD episodes, on the other hand, occur during REM sleep, and people frequently retain vivid memories of their dreams.

3. Some nocturnal seizures can resemble the movements and behaviors observed in RBD. Seizures, on the other hand, usually begin abruptly and may be accompanied by other symptoms such as incontinence or tongue biting. To distinguish between RBD and seizure disorders, a full medical assessment is required, which may include a sleep study and potentially an EEG.

4. Obstructive Sleep Apnea (OSA): While OSA is typically defined as breathing disruptions during sleep, it can also result in fragmented sleep and awakenings. People with OSA may twitch or thrash in reaction to choking feelings. However, the fundamental issue with OSA is airway obstruction, not the dream enactment actions observed in RBD.

Recognizing these discrepancies is critical for proper diagnosis and therapy. A sleep expert can do a comprehensive sleep study called polysomnography to monitor sleep patterns, muscle activity, and brain waves. This investigation aids in distinguishing RBD from other disorders and validating the diagnosis.

Chapter 3

The Possibility of Cure

One of the most urgent problems about REM Sleep Behavior Disorder (RBD) is whether it is curable. Currently, the medical profession lacks a definite cure for RBD. However, tremendous progress has been made in understanding the disease and treating its symptoms.

RBD is a neurological condition that impairs the proper functioning of REM sleep. During REM sleep, the brain often sends messages inhibiting muscular movement, thereby paralyzing the body and preventing it from acting out dreams. RBD causes this inhibition to fail, resulting in potentially harmful physical activities during sleep.

Researchers have found numerous possible causes of RBD. These include neurodegenerative disorders like

Parkinson's disease and Lewy body dementia. In fact, RBD is typically seen as one of the first signs of these disorders. Other possible reasons include some drugs, notably antidepressants, and withdrawal from alcohol or sedatives.

Given its link to neurological problems, treating RBD frequently entails addressing the underlying disease. For example, in Parkinson's disease patients, managing Parkinson's progression can assist lower the intensity of RBD symptoms. However, for many, the focus is still on symptom management rather than a total cure.

Breakthrough and ongoing research

While there is no cure for RBD, continuing research is offering insight into prospective therapies and strategies for better managing the disorder. Scientists and medical experts are working relentlessly to better understand the processes that cause RBD and discover solutions.

1. Pharmacological Treatments: Medications remain the major method of treating RBD symptoms. Melatonin and clonazepam are the most widely utilized medications. Melatonin, a hormone that governs sleep wake cycles, is commonly utilized due to its low side effects and typically good tolerance. Clonazepam, a benzodiazepine, is useful in lowering aggressive behavior but can lead to dependence and other negative effects. Researchers are looking at other drugs that may provide similar advantages without the downsides.

2. Neuroprotective medicines: Given the association between RBD and neurodegenerative disorders, several researchers are looking into medicines that might protect or repair neurons. These neuroprotective medicines try to reduce or stop the course of illnesses such as Parkinson's, perhaps alleviating RBD symptoms as well. While this study is still in its early phases, it shows promise for future treatments.

3. Genetic Studies: Genetic research is very important in understanding RBD. Scientists want to pinpoint

particular genes that contribute to RBD by researching the genetic composition of those who have it. This insight may lead to tailored medicines that address the underlying causes of RBD.

4. Brain Stimulation: Potential therapies for RBD include transcranial magnetic stimulation (TMS) and deep brain stimulation (DBS). These techniques include stimulating particular parts of the brain to enhance neurological function. While these approaches are largely employed to treat depression and Parkinson's disease, there is optimism that they will also assist those with RBD.

5. Lifestyle and Behavioral therapy: In addition to drugs, lifestyle adjustments, and behavioral therapy can be very effective in controlling RBD. Improving sleep hygiene, lowering stress, and providing a safe sleeping environment can all help reduce the risk of injury during RBD episodes. Cognitive behavioral therapy (CBT) and other treatment techniques are also being investigated to

assist people deal with the emotional and psychological effects of the condition.

Remission and Management.

While a definitive treatment for RBD is still elusive, there are several instances of people who have discovered strategies to manage their symptoms and live happy lives. These tales give hope and inspiration to people living with RBD and their loved ones.

1. Managing Medication: One person with RBD experienced great alleviation with a combination of melatonin and clonazepam. Working closely with their doctor to alter doses and check side effects allowed them to lessen the frequency and intensity of their bouts. This helped them sleep better and wake up feeling more refreshed.

2. Creating a Safe Sleep Environment: Another person took proactive efforts to ensure a safe sleep environment. They put cushioning around the bed and removed any

sharp or harsh things from the room. These modifications greatly lowered the risk of harm during RBD episodes, giving them and their spouse peace of mind.

3. Lifestyle Changes: Some people have discovered that changing their lifestyle can help them manage their RBD symptoms significantly. This includes sticking to a consistent sleep schedule, avoiding alcohol and caffeine before bedtime, and practicing relaxation techniques such as meditation or deep breathing exercises. These changes helped one person minimize the severity of their episodes and enhance their overall sleep quality.

4. Support Groups and Therapy: Emotional support is an important part of controlling RBD. Joining a support group or seeking therapy might allow people to share their experiences and learn from one another. One individual discovered that speaking with people who knew their difficulties made them feel less alone and more empowered to manage their illness.

5. Ongoing Research Participation: Some RBD patients have found hope by participating in clinical trials and research projects. By contributing to scientific knowledge and testing novel treatments, people not only obtain access to cutting edge medicines but also help pave the road for future advances in RBD therapy.

While these anecdotes demonstrate the tenacity and adaptation of persons living with RBD, they also emphasize the significance of ongoing research and medical advances. Each step forward takes us closer to more effective treatments and, eventually, cures.

Chapter 4

Managing and Stopping REM Behavior Disorder

Managing REM Sleep Behavior Disorder (RBD) frequently begins with medicinal therapies. Medications can be quite successful at lowering the frequency and severity of RBD episodes. Clonazepam and melatonin are the most typically given drugs for RBD.

Clonazepam, a benzodiazepine, has been used for many years to treat RBD. It works by relaxing the nervous system and decreasing the possibility of physical activity during REM sleep. Clonazepam is often used before bedtime and has been shown to greatly reduce the aggressive behaviors associated with RBD. However, clonazepam has possible adverse effects such as sleepiness, dizziness, and the possibility of dependency, therefore it should only be used under constant medical supervision.

Melatonin is a hormone that affects sleep and waking cycles. It has fewer negative effects than clonazepam and is frequently suggested as the first line therapy. Melatonin improves sleep quality and can lessen the number of RBD episodes. It is typically well tolerated and can be an effective long term treatment.

Other medicines, in addition to those listed above, may be recommended based on the needs of each patient. Antidepressants that influence serotonin levels, for example, might assist at times but can potentially increase symptoms in others. Working with a sleep specialist is critical for determining the most effective drug and dose.

Beyond drugs, various treatments can be effective. Cognitive behavioral therapy (CBT) is one method for helping patients manage stress and anxiety, which can contribute to RBD symptoms. CBT can teach coping methods and relaxation techniques to improve sleep hygiene and minimize the number of episodes.

Behavioral Strategies and Lifestyle Changes

While drugs are crucial, behavioral interventions and lifestyle adjustments can also help manage RBD. Creating a consistent nighttime routine and practicing excellent sleep hygiene are essential stages.

Stress management is critical since stress can worsen RBD symptoms. Mindfulness meditation, yoga, and deep breathing exercises can all help you relax before bedtime. Creating a peaceful pre sleep ritual, such as reading a book, having a warm bath, or listening to soothing music, helps alert the body that it is time to unwind.

Avoiding triggers is another critical tactic. This includes minimizing alcohol and caffeine consumption, particularly in the hours before bedtime. Both drugs can alter sleep patterns and raise the risk of RBD episodes.

Furthermore, several drugs might interfere with sleep, therefore it is critical to examine all medications with a healthcare specialist to see which ones may be contributing to RBD.

Regular exercise might also be helpful. Physical activity regulates the sleep wake cycle and can lower stress levels. However, it is vital to avoid strenuous activity close to sleep because it may stimulate rather than calm. Aim for moderate activity early in the day to gain the sleep advantages without interrupting your nightly sleep.

Creating A Safe Sleep Environment

One of the most practical tasks in controlling RBD is to create a safe sleeping environment. Because RBD can cause potentially harmful actions while sleeping, making the bedroom a safe environment is crucial.

Remove any sharp objects and anything else that might cause damage during an incident. This may entail relocating furniture with sharp edges, fastening lights, and removing breakable items from the bedside table. Padding the floor surrounding the bed can also assist in lessening the likelihood of damage if the individual falls out of bed.

Consider the bed itself. Using a low bed or laying the mattress on the floor can help prevent falls. Installing bed rails with cushioning can also give another degree of protection. Additionally, ensuring that the windows and doors are locked will keep the individual from accidentally exiting the bedroom and straying into potentially harmful locations.

Protecting bed companions is also essential. This may include sleeping in separate beds or even rooms if required. If the episodes are light, putting a barrier between couples or using a weighted blanket might assist in reducing the impact of any movements during sleep.

The Role of Diet and Exercise

Diet and exercise can have a major influence on sleep quality and the treatment of RBD symptoms. A balanced diet rich in nutrients enhances general health and well being, which leads to better sleep.

Certain meals and minerals are proven to promote sleep. For example, meals high in tryptophan, such as turkey, eggs, and nuts, can assist boost the synthesis of melatonin and serotonin, which regulate sleep. Magnesium rich foods, such as leafy greens, bananas, and almonds, might help you relax and sleep better.

Staying hydrated is crucial, but avoid drinking big amounts of fluids close to bedtime to lessen the possibility of waking up throughout the night. Limiting coffee and alcohol consumption is critical since both can interfere with sleep. Instead, try herbal teas or warm milk in the evening for a relaxing effect.

Regular physical activity promotes a healthy sleep/wake cycle. Exercise can help reduce tension and worry, which are typical causes of RBD episodes. Moderate aerobic activity, such as walking, swimming, or cycling, for at least 30 minutes most days of the week will help you sleep better. Strength and flexibility activities, such as yoga or Pilates, might also be useful.

It's crucial to remember that exercise should be done at the appropriate time of day. Vigorous activity too close to bedtime might be stimulating and make it difficult to fall asleep. Try to finish any strenuous workouts at least a couple hours before bedtime. In contrast, gentle stretching or yoga in the evening can help the body relax and prepare for sleep.

Chapter 5

Understanding the Differences Between RBD and Sleepwalking

To comprehend the distinctions between REM Sleep Behavior Disorder (RBD) and sleepwalking, it is necessary to examine the processes underlying each disorder. Both include aberrant sleep activities, but they occur at various periods of the sleep cycle and are triggered by distinct underlying mechanisms.

REM Sleep Behavior Disorder (RBD) develops during the REM (Rapid Eye Movement) period of sleep, when most dreams occur. Normally, during REM sleep, the brain releases signals that stop muscular movement, thereby paralyzing the body and preventing it from acting out dreams. In people with RBD, this paralysis is partial or absent, allowing them to physically act out their dreams, such as kicking, punching, or even jumping out of bed. The dreams in RBD are frequently vivid and powerful, and the activities are usually consistent with the dream content.

Sleepwalking (somnambulism) occurs during non REM (NREM) sleep, namely during the deep sleep periods (stages 3 and 4). During these stages, the brain is not actively paralyzing the muscles, but it is also not in a position to experience complex dreams. Sleepwalking is a partial waking from deep sleep in which the individual shows actions such as sitting up in bed, walking around, completing ordinary tasks, or even leaving the house. Sleepwalkers, unlike RBD, frequently have no recall of their acts upon waking, and their behaviors are more automatic and less coordinated than those observed in RBD.

Symptoms and Behaviors

When comparing RBD to sleepwalking, it is evident that each illness has unique symptoms and activities.

Understanding these distinctions can aid in recognizing and managing illnesses more effectively.

Symptoms of RBD:

- Vivid Dream Enactment: RBD is distinguished by the physical enactment of vivid, often violent, dreams. This can entail striking, kicking, or even getting out of bed to participate in complex actions that correspond to the dream material.
- Awareness: People with RBD frequently recall their dreams and the acts they took during the episodes, which distinguishes them from sleepwalkers.
- RBD episodes occur during REM sleep, usually in the second half of the night when REM sleep is most prominent.

Symptoms of Sleepwalking:

- Sleepwalking activities are more automatic than deliberate. They can include sitting up in bed, going about, eating, and even driving, but the motions are often sloppy and uncoordinated.

- Lack of Awareness: Sleepwalkers are often unaware of their activities and have little to no recall of the incident when they wake up.
- Sleepwalking occurs during deep NREM sleep, particularly in the first third of the night when deep sleep phases are most prevalent.

These changes in symptoms and behaviors are crucial for differentiating between the two illnesses. RBD is distinguished by dream enactment with knowledge of the incident, whereas sleepwalking involves non purposeful, automatic activities with no memory of the occurrence.

Treatment Strategies for Each Disorder

The treatment techniques for RBD and sleepwalking differ greatly, reflecting their distinct causes and symptoms.

Treatment of RBD:
- Medications: As described in earlier chapters, clonazepam and melatonin are often used to treat

RBD. These drugs assist in lowering the frequency and severity of dream enactment activities by encouraging muscular relaxation and regulating sleep cycles.

- Creating a Safe Sleep Environment: Providing a safe sleeping environment is critical for those with RBD. This involves removing sharp objects, cushioning furniture, and potentially installing bed rails to avoid falls.

- Behavioral Therapies: Cognitive behavioral therapy (CBT) and stress management approaches may be effective. RBD symptoms can be managed by reducing stress and anxiety with relaxation techniques, meditation, and consistent sleep patterns.

Treatment for Sleep Walking:

- Sleep Hygiene: Improving sleep hygiene is a fundamental strategy for managing sleepwalking. This includes adhering to a consistent sleep schedule, developing a calming nighttime ritual, and establishing a pleasant sleeping environment.

- Safety precautions: As with RBD, safety is crucial. This might involve locking windows and doors, removing harmful objects, and potentially installing alarms to notify family members if the sleepwalker exits the bed.

- Addressing Underlying Conditions: Sleepwalking can be caused by sleep apnea, restless leg syndrome, or certain drugs. Treating these diseases can minimize the number of sleepwalking occurrences.

- Medications: In certain circumstances, benzodiazepines or antidepressants may be administered to assist treat sleepwalking, particularly if the episodes are frequent or severe.

Both RBD and sleepwalking have a substantial influence on the lives of individuals affected and their families. Understanding the variations in their causes, symptoms, and therapies can result in more effective management and higher quality of life.

Connecting the Dots:

Managing RBD and sleepwalking necessitates a comprehensive strategy that includes both medicinal and lifestyle changes. While drugs and treatments are helpful, lifestyle adjustments and safety precautions are also necessary to ensure the well being of those suffering from these sleep disorders.

Education and Support: Educating patients and their families on the nature of these diseases is critical. Understanding the triggers, symptoms, and treatments can help people make proactive efforts to manage their disease. Support groups and therapy can also offer emotional and practical guidance.

Regular Monitoring: Regular follow ups with healthcare providers are required to assess the efficacy of therapy and make appropriate modifications. This may include sleep tests, a sleep diary, and regular evaluations of any changes in symptoms or behaviors.

Collaborative Care: A team approach that includes sleep experts, neurologists, and mental health doctors can provide complete care. Each professional can offer their skills to create a treatment plan that is suited to the patient's specific needs.

Maintaining overall health is critical, which includes eating a well balanced diet, exercising regularly, and managing stress. Healthy lifestyle choices can increase sleep quality while decreasing the frequency of RBD and sleepwalking episodes.

Individuals suffering from RBD and sleepwalking can effectively manage their symptoms and live safer, happier lives by taking a complete and integrated strategy. Understanding the unique features and treatment options for each problem is the first step toward improving sleep quality and general well being.

Chapter 6

Triggers and Risk Factors for RBD

Understanding what causes REM Sleep Behavior Disorder (RBD) and recognizing the risk factors might assist manage and perhaps prevent its occurrence. This section digs into the different factors that lead to the development of RBD, including genetic predispositions, environmental impacts, and the links to psychological and physical health.

Genetic predispositions

Genetics can significantly influence the probability of getting RBD. While the study continues, there is evidence that RBD can run in families, indicating a genetic component. Certain genes may influence the brain circuits that control REM sleep and muscular atonia (the typical paralysis that happens during REM sleep), rendering certain people more vulnerable to RBD.

Family History: If a close family has RBD or another associated neurological disorder, such as Parkinson's disease, the chance of acquiring RBD rises. This familial relationship implies that inherited genetic elements may contribute to the illness.

Genetic Mutations: Certain genetic mutations have been connected to RBD. These mutations can impair the generation or function of proteins required for appropriate sleep architecture and muscle atonia during REM sleep. For example, mutations in the SNCA gene, which produces alpha synuclein (a protein seen in Parkinson's disease and Lewy body dementia), have been linked to RBD.

Environmental and Lifestyle Factors

Aside from genetics, a variety of environmental and lifestyle variables might impact the onset and progression of RBD. These variables can combine with genetic predispositions to either increase or reduce the risk.

Drugs and Substances: Some drugs, particularly those that impact the central nervous system, can cause or exacerbate RBD. Antidepressants, particularly selective serotonin reuptake inhibitors (SSRIs) and serotonin norepinephrine reuptake inhibitors (SNRIs), have been linked to increased RBD symptoms. Furthermore, substances such as alcohol and recreational drugs can alter regular sleep patterns, contributing to RBD.

Stress and Trauma: Excessive stress or traumatic situations can significantly impair sleep. Chronic stress can change the balance of neurotransmitters in the brain, influencing sleep architecture and increasing the risk of RBD. Traumatic brain injuries and post traumatic stress disorder (PTSD) are also substantial risk factors because they can impair normal brain functioning associated with sleep.

Sleep Deprivation: A lack of enough sleep might worsen RBD symptoms. Sleep deprivation increases the need for REM sleep, which might result in more intense and frequent REM phases, increasing the likelihood of dream enactment actions.

Lifestyle Choices: Poor eating habits, lack of exercise, and inconsistent sleep schedules can all contribute to the development of RBD. Maintaining a nutritious diet, participating in regular physical activity, and adhering to a normal sleep schedule can all assist in reducing some of these risks.

Psychological and Physical Health Connections

The relationship between psychological and physical health and RBD is considerable. Several illnesses can cause or exacerbate RBD symptoms, emphasizing the significance of a comprehensive approach to health.

There is a well documented link between RBD and neurodegenerative illnesses, including Parkinson's disease and Lewy body dementia. RBD frequently precedes these illnesses by several years, acting as an early warning signal. This relationship emphasizes the significance of tracking and controlling RBD symptoms, which might suggest underlying neurodegenerative processes.

Anxiety, depression, and other mental health issues are widespread among people with RBD. These factors can interrupt typical sleep patterns and increase the risk of REM sleep without atonia. RBD symptoms can be reduced with effective mental health care, which includes therapy, medication, and lifestyle modifications.

Chronic conditions, such as diabetes, cardiovascular disease, and respiratory problems, can all have an influence on sleep quality and contribute to RBD. Managing these disorders via proper medical care and lifestyle changes is critical to lowering RBD risk.

Hormonal Changes: Hormonal variations, particularly in women, can disrupt sleep patterns and raise the risk of

RBD. For example, menopause is linked to changes in sleep architecture, which might predispose women to sleep disorders such as RBD.

Integrating Knowledge into Management Strategies.

Understanding the causes and risk factors of RBD is the first step toward successful therapy. By addressing these variables, individuals can make proactive efforts to minimize their risk and better manage symptoms.

Genetic Counseling: Genetic counseling might be beneficial for people who have a family history of RBD or other neurological disorders. Understanding one's genetic propensity enables early surveillance and intervention.

Medication Review: A regular medication review with a healthcare professional is essential, especially if symptoms of RBD arise after starting a new drug. Adjusting doses or switching to different therapies can help to reduce the risk.

Stress Management: Using stress management strategies like mindfulness, meditation, and yoga can greatly improve sleep quality and alleviate RBD symptoms. Cognitive behavioral therapy (CBT) can also help to manage stress and anxiety.

Healthy Lifestyle Choices: Adopting a healthy lifestyle that includes a balanced diet, frequent exercise, and a consistent sleep pattern is essential. Avoiding alcohol and recreational drugs, as well as creating a relaxing and favorable sleep environment, can all assist with RBD management.

Regular Medical Checkups: Regular health screenings can aid in the identification and management of chronic diseases that may contribute to RBD. Early diagnosis and treatment of neurological illnesses, mental health issues, and other chronic diseases is critical for good health and sleep quality.

Chapter 7

When Does RBD Start

Understanding when Rapid Eye Movement (REM) Sleep Behavior Disorder (RBD) usually starts is critical for early detection and treatment. This section looks at the normal age of onset, early warning indicators in various age groups, and probable gender variations in frequency and symptoms.

Typical age of onset

RBD can appear at any age, however there are certain tendencies about when it usually starts. While the illness can arise in infancy or adolescence, it usually appears later in life, with an average age of occurrence ranging from the late 50s to early 70s. However, it is important to remember that individual experiences differ, and RBD might emerge sooner or later based on variables such as heredity, lifestyle, and underlying health issues.

Early Warning Signs for Various Age Groups

Childhood and Adolescence:

In rare circumstances, RBD can manifest in infancy or adolescence. Early indications of RBD in these age ranges might include:

- Violent or Disruptive Sleep: Parents may observe bouts of strong activity or vocalizations while their kid sleeps, such as kicking, punching, or screaming.
- Sleep Disturbances: Children with RBD may wake up often during the night, complain of nightmares, or have disrupted sleep.
- Daytime Behavioral Changes: Daytime symptoms such as impatience, mood swings, or difficulties focusing may suggest interrupted sleep patterns caused by RBD.

Adults:

RBD is most typically diagnosed in adults, especially in midlife and later. Adults may exhibit the following early warning signs:

- Dream Enactment Behaviors: Adults with RBD may physically act out their dreams while sleeping, causing injury or disrupting their sleep environment.
- Sleep related injuries: Reports of falls, bruising, or injuries experienced while sleeping may indicate RBD.
- Bed Partner Observations: Partners or family members may observe strange activities while sleeping, such as kicking, punching, or vocalizations, necessitating more examination.

Elderly Population:

RBD prevalence rises with age, especially among elderly persons. Early indications of RBD in the elderly might include:

- Increased Symptom Frequency: Older folks may have more frequent and acute dream enactment activities than younger people.
- Memory Disturbances: Some people may have memory lapses or disorientation upon awakening, indicating cognitive involvement.
- Motor Symptoms: Other motor symptoms, such as tremors or stiffness, may indicate a relationship between RBD and neurodegenerative diseases like Parkinson's.

Gender Differences in RBD Prevalence and Symptoms.

While RBD can affect people of both genders, the incidence and symptom presentation may differ between men and women.

RBD appears to be more frequent in men than in women, with research indicating a greater frequency among men. However, the causes of this gender discrepancy are not well understood and may entail a complicated interplay of biological, genetic, and environmental variables.

Symptom Presentation: While the primary symptoms of RBD are comparable across genders, there may be differences in how they appear or are reported. For example, some studies imply that men may engage in more aggressive or violent dream enactment practices than women. Furthermore, hormonal variations in women, such as those associated with menstruation or menopause, might affect the intensity or frequency of RBD symptoms.

Integrating Knowledge into Early Intervention.

Recognizing the age at the beginning and early warning indications of RBD is critical for proper intervention and therapy. Individuals and their healthcare professionals may successfully treat RBD by recognizing when it normally develops and being aware of possible warning flags at various periods of life.

Early Screening: Healthcare practitioners should consider screening for RBD in those who have suggestive symptoms, especially during regular health exams or sleep disruption examinations.

Education and Awareness: Educating individuals and their families about the signs and symptoms of RBD can help encourage early detection and timely medical examination and treatment.

Individuals at increased risk of RBD, such as those with a family history of the illness or other neurodegenerative disorders, require regular monitoring and follow up consultations with healthcare specialists to ensure early identification and management.

Individualized Care: Tailoring therapies to meet the particular requirements and problems of people with RBD, taking into consideration age, gender, and other health conditions, can enhance results and quality of life.

Chapter 8

The Causes of Acting Out Dreams

Understanding the underlying reasons for dreams acting in Rapid Eye Movement (REM) Sleep Behavior Disorder (RBD) is critical for successful treatment and intervention. This section examines the neurological bases of RBD, how brain functions differ in RBD patients, and how neurodegenerative illnesses affect dream enactment behaviors.

Neurological Foundations of RBD

RBD is defined by the lack of normal muscular atonia during REM sleep, which results in the development of dream enactment activities. The fundamental neurological issue linked with RBD is impairment in the brain networks that regulate REM sleep and muscular control. RBD involves many critical parts of the brain:

The brainstem regulates sleep wake cycles and coordinates muscle activity during sleep. RBD is hypothesized to be caused by dysfunction in certain nuclei in the brainstem, notably those responsible for REM sleep production and muscular atonia.

The hypothalamus controls a variety of physiological functions, including sleep and wakefulness. Disruptions in hypothalamic function may affect REM sleep pathways, contributing to the emergence of RBD symptoms.

Limbic System: The limbic system, which includes components like the amygdala and hippocampus, is responsible for emotional processing and memory creation. Abnormalities in limbic system function may influence the content and intensity of dreams during REM sleep, potentially leading to more vivid and emotionally charged dream enactment activities in RBD.

How Brain Functions Differ in RBD Patients

Research on the neurobiology of RBD has found substantial changes in brain functions and structures between persons with and without the disorder:

Functional Brain Imaging: Researchers have used techniques such as functional magnetic resonance imaging (fMRI) to identify changes in brain activity patterns during REM sleep in people with RBD. These alterations frequently involve parts of the brain responsible for motor control, emotion processing, and self awareness, emphasizing the intricate interaction of neuronal circuits implicated in RBD symptoms.

Structural Brain Changes: Structural neuroimaging studies have revealed changes in brain structure, notably in areas involved in REM sleep control and motor function, in RBD patients. These structural abnormalities might indicate underlying neurodegenerative processes or changes in brain connections associated with RBD disease.

Neurotransmitter Imbalance: RBD has been linked to dysregulation of neurotransmitter systems such as serotonin, dopamine, and noradrenaline. Imbalances in these neurotransmitters can alter the delicate balance of alertness and muscle atonia during REM sleep, resulting in dream enactment activities.

The impact of neurodegenerative diseases.

RBD is frequently seen as a prodromal or early stage of neurodegenerative disorders such as Parkinson's disease and Lewy body dementia. The link between RBD and neurodegeneration emphasizes the larger consequences of dream enactment behaviors:

RBD may serve as a prognostic sign for the development of neurodegenerative disorders since longitudinal studies have shown a high conversion rate from isolated RBD to Parkinson's disease or dementia with Lewy bodies over time. Monitoring people with RBD for the appearance of new neurological symptoms is critical for early discovery and treatment.

RBD and neurodegenerative illnesses have identical pathophysiological processes, including the buildup of aberrant protein aggregates such as alpha synuclein. These common clinical traits point to overlapping disease mechanisms and possible treatment options for both RBD and related neurodegenerative disorders.

Management Implications: Understanding the relationship between RBD and neurodegeneration has significant implications for disease management and therapy. Strategies focused on delaying disease progression and preserving cognitive function may assist people with RBD, especially those who are more likely to acquire neurodegenerative disorders.

Integrating knowledge into treatment approaches.

Understanding the reasons for acting out dreams in RBD allows for the creation of tailored treatment approaches:

Pharmacological Interventions: Medications that target neurotransmitter systems involved in RBD, such as clonazepam and melatonin, can assist afflicted people relieve symptoms and enhance their sleep quality.

Non pharmacological Therapies: Behavioral strategies such as sleep hygiene education, cognitive behavioral therapy for insomnia (CBT I), and relaxation methods can supplement pharmaceutical treatments and improve overall treatment results.

Disease modifying medicines: Emerging medicines that attempt to slow or stop the course of neurodegenerative disorders may offer promise for avoiding or delaying the onset of RBD symptoms and associated neurodegeneration.

Chapter 9

Understanding the Signs of RBD

Diagnosing Rapid Eye Movement (REM) Sleep Behavior Disorder (RBD) is critical for early intervention and treatment. This section gives a complete approach to recognizing RBD, including step by step indicators to look for, diagnostic tests and sleep studies used in diagnosis, and recommendations on when to seek professional treatment.

How to Identify RBD: A Step by Step Guide

Recognizing the signs and symptoms of RBD is the first step toward making an accurate diagnosis. Here's a step by step approach for determining RBD:

1. Pay attention to any odd sleep activities, such as kicking, hitting, shouting, or writhing. These actions

frequently occur during REM sleep and might be reported by a bedmate or family member.

2. Document Frequency and Severity: Keep track of how frequently these behaviors occur and how they affect sleep quality and daily functioning. Frequent or severe instances of dream enactment actions may necessitate additional examination.

3. Note Dream Content: Ask the person experiencing symptoms to recount their dreams or nightmares. RBD related dreams frequently feature dramatic, vivid, and action packed scenes that may elicit bodily reactions while sleeping.

4. Consider Risk Factors: Look for any underlying medical problems or drugs that might predispose people to RBD, such as neurodegenerative illnesses, antidepressants, or certain mental disorders.

5. Examine Daytime Symptoms: Inquire about any daytime symptoms related to interrupted sleep, such as

increased daytime drowsiness, exhaustion, irritability, or memory problems. These symptoms may suggest underlying sleep problems, such as RBD.

Diagnostic Tests and Sleep Studies

RBD is frequently diagnosed using a combination of clinical examination and specialist sleep testing. The following are the key diagnostic tests and sleep studies used to diagnose RBD:

1. Clinical Evaluation: A complete medical history and physical examination are required to identify potential risk factors and rule out other sleep disorders or other diseases that may resemble RBD.

2. Polysomnography (PSG) is the gold standard diagnostic test for RBD. Individuals are monitored nightly in a sleep laboratory for abnormalities in REM sleep and accompanying motor activities.

3. Video Polysomnography (VPSG) combines standard PSG with video surveillance to capture and document dream enactment activities in real time, giving new diagnostic information and verifying the existence of RBD.

4. Multiple Sleep Latency Test (MSLT): The MSLT may be used to examine daytime drowsiness and rule out other causes of excessive daytime sleepiness, such as narcolepsy, which can coexist with RBD.

When to Seek Professional Help:

Knowing when to seek professional help for suspected RBD is critical for getting an accurate diagnosis and receiving the right therapy. Here are some indicators that it's time to contact a healthcare provider:

1. Persistent or Severe Symptoms: If dream enactment actions occur regularly, interrupt sleep, or represent a danger of damage to the individual or others, quick medical attention is recommended.

2. Concerns about Safety: If a bed partner or family member expresses worry about a person's safety as a result of their sleeping habits, they should seek medical attention immediately.

3. Daytime Impairment: Excessive daytime drowsiness, weariness, irritability, memory difficulties, or other daytime symptoms indicating interrupted sleep should be evaluated by a healthcare practitioner.

4. Individuals with established risk factors for RBD, such as a family history of the illness or underlying neurological disorders, should consult with a healthcare physician, even if they are not experiencing symptoms.

Chapter 10

Communicating and Living with Someone with RBD

Living with someone suffering from Rapid Eye Movement (REM) Sleep Behavior Disorder (RBD) can bring unique issues for both the affected person and their loved ones. This section delves into effective communication tactics, the value of creating a supportive environment, coping mechanisms for families and caregivers, and real life examples of families prospering despite RBD issues.

Effective Communication Strategies

Communication is essential for negotiating the complications of living with RBD. Here are some successful communication tactics for dealing with someone who has RBD:

1. Open and Honest Dialogue: Create an environment in which both parties feel free to communicate their views, worries, and feelings concerning RBD related issues.

2. Active listening is paying full attention to the person speaking, empathizing with their experiences, and validating their sentiments without judgment or criticism.

3. Clarity and Consistency: When discussing RBD related subjects, use clear and unambiguous language to avoid ambiguity or confusion. Maintain consistency in communication to avoid misconceptions.

4. Respect Boundaries: Recognize the individual's need for privacy and personal space, particularly during bouts of RBD related behavior. Avoid asking invasive questions or doing acts that may heighten feelings of discomfort or vulnerability.

5. Collaborative Problem Solving entails approaching issues and disputes collectively, seeking mutually acceptable solutions and compromises that promote both sides' well being.

Creating a supportive environment

Creating a supportive atmosphere is critical for improving the physical and emotional well being of people with RBD. Here are some ideas for creating a helpful environment.

1. Safe Sleep Environment: Make sure the sleep environment is safe and conducive to peaceful sleep, and remove any possible dangers such as sharp items, hard surfaces, or barriers that might represent a risk during RBD episodes.

2. Structured nighttime ritual: Create a consistent nighttime ritual that encourages relaxation and prepares the individual for sleep. Incorporate calming hobbies like

reading, listening to relaxing music, or practicing relaxation methods.

3. Emotional Support: Provide emotional support and comfort to the RBD patient, acknowledging their difficulties and validating their experiences. Offer a listening ear and a shoulder to lean on at trying times.

4. Education and Awareness: Inform family members, caregivers, and others in the home about RBD, including its symptoms, causes, and treatment options. Increase knowledge and understanding in order to build empathy and support within the home.

Coping Strategies for Family and Caregivers

Caring for someone with RBD may be both emotionally and physically exhausting. Here are some coping strategies for family members and caregivers:

1. Prioritize self care and well being to avoid burnout and remain resilient in the midst of caring problems.

Take pauses, seek help from others, and do things that encourage relaxation and stress alleviation.

2. Seeking Support: For help and encouragement, contact support groups, internet forums, or professional counseling services. Connecting with people who are going through similar situations may give affirmation, insight, and practical help.

3. Setting Realistic Expectations: Recognize that caring for someone with RBD may include ups and downs, setbacks, and uncertainty. Set reasonable goals for yourself and the person with RBD, recognizing limitations and enjoying minor accomplishments along the way.

4. Flexibility and Adaptability: Be adaptive in your approach to caring, altering routines, techniques, and expectations as needed to account for changing circumstances and developing needs.

Living with someone with RBD needs patience, understanding, and the ability to adjust to changing situations. Families may overcome the challenges of RBD with grace and tenacity by using good communication skills, creating a supportive atmosphere, practicing self care, and gaining inspiration from real life examples of resilience. Together, they can construct a road ahead that values optimism, compassion, and the power of human connection in overcoming adversity.

Chapter 11

Thriving Regardless of RBD, Practical Tips for a Productive Life

Living with Rapid Eye Movement (REM) Sleep Behavior Disorder (RBD) brings unique obstacles, but with the appropriate techniques in place, you may live a meaningful and productive life. This section delves into practical recommendations for balancing work, social life, and RBD, stress management and mental health, and long term planning and adaption techniques for thriving in the face of RBD issues.

Balancing Work, Social Life, and RBD.

Maintaining a work life balance while also controlling RBD is critical for general well being and productivity. Here are some practical ways to achieve balance:

1. Flexible Work Arrangements: Consider flexible work arrangements, such as telecommuting or modifying work hours, to suit the unexpected nature of RBD symptoms.

2. Open Communication with Employers: Inform employers or supervisors about your health and any adjustments or assistance required to execute work tasks efficiently. Establishing a supportive work environment can reduce stress and aid in the treatment of RBD.

3. Prioritize Self Care: Set aside time for relaxation, exercise, and activities that improve physical and mental well being. Prioritizing self care can help relieve stress and improve overall sleep quality.

4. Social Support: Build a network of friends, family members, or support groups that understand and empathize with your RBD journey. Sharing your experiences and seeking help from others can give emotional affirmation and encouragement.

Stress Management and Mental Health

Managing stress and preserving mental health are critical components of dealing with RBD. Here are some ways to manage stress and boost mental health:

1. Stress Reduction Techniques: Deep breathing exercises, meditation, yoga, or progressive muscle relaxation can all help to calm the mind and body during stressful or anxious situations.

2. Healthy Lifestyle Choices: Practice healthy lifestyle habits such as regular exercise, balanced eating, proper sleep hygiene, and abstaining from alcohol, caffeine, and nicotine, which can aggravate RBD symptoms and add to stress.

3. Seeking Professional Help: Talk to a therapist or counselor who specializes in sleep problems or anxiety management. Professional assistance can give useful coping methods and emotional support.

4. Mindfulness and Acceptance: Use mindfulness and acceptance strategies to build resilience and acceptance of the obstacles presented by RBD. Acceptance can assist minimize ruminating and discomfort caused by RBD related symptoms.

Long term Planning and Adaptation Strategies.

Maintaining a sense of control and autonomy requires long term planning and adaptation to RBD problems. Below are some long term planning and adaption strategies:

1. Financial Planning: Plan for future financial stability by saving money, investing in insurance, and investigating disability benefits or accommodations if necessary due to RBD related restrictions.

2. Life Transitions: Anticipate and plan for important life transitions, such as retirement or changes in living arrangements, taking into account the impact of RBD on everyday functioning and lifestyle choices.

3. Technology and Assistive Equipment: Look into technology solutions and assistive equipment that can help manage RBD symptoms, such as sleep tracking applications, smart home gadgets, and safety alerts to prevent harm during sleep disruptions.

4. Advocacy and Education: Help raise awareness and knowledge of RBD in the community, healthcare system, and workplace. Educating people about RBD can help to eliminate stigma, increase empathy, and improve access to support and services.

Conclusion

As our understanding of Rapid Eye Movement (REM) Sleep Behavior Disorder (RBD) grows, so does our approach to research, treatment, and support for people living with it. In this section, we will look at the future of RBD research and therapy, provide some concluding comments and encouragement to individuals living with RBD, and suggest resources and support networks for more help.

The Future of RBD Research and Treatment.

The area of RBD research is quickly evolving, with continuing efforts aimed at expanding our understanding of the underlying processes, developing new treatment modalities, and enhancing the quality of life for those affected by RBD. Future studies should focus on several crucial topics, including:

1. Neurological Mechanisms: Research the neurological mechanisms that underpin RBD in order to better understand its pathogenesis and find possible targets for treatments.

2. Genetic and Environmental variables: Investigating the role of genetic predispositions and environmental variables in the development and progression of RBD in order to provide tailored treatment strategies.

3. Clinical trials are conducted to assess the safety and efficacy of innovative treatment interventions such as pharmaceutical drugs, behavioral therapies, and neurostimulation methods.

4. Long Term results: Longitudinal studies examine the long term results and prognosis of RBD patients, including the risk of acquiring neurodegenerative disorders such as Parkinson's disease and Lewy body dementia.

By conducting rigorous scientific research and cooperation, we can create more effective treatment techniques and enhance the quality of life for those living with RBD.

Embracing Life with RBD: Final Thoughts and Encouragements

Living with RBD might provide unique obstacles, but remember that you are not alone. With the correct support, tools, and coping skills, it is possible to have a productive and meaningful life despite the challenges given by this sleep illness. Here are some last thoughts and words of encouragement for individuals living with RBD.

1. You Are Resilient: Despite the difficulties of RBD, you have demonstrated tremendous resilience in navigating the ups and downs of the illness. Your strength and endurance demonstrate your inner resilience and resolve.

2. Seek Support: Do not be afraid to seek help from friends, family, healthcare experts, or support groups. Surround yourself with individuals who understand and empathize with your situation, and don't be hesitant to seek assistance when required.

3. Focus on What You Can Control: While living with RBD can be difficult, focus on what you can change, such as adopting good lifestyle choices, getting therapy and support, and practicing self care.

4. Stay Informed: Learn about the most recent research, treatment choices, and support services for people with RBD. Knowledge is power, and staying educated may help you make better decisions regarding your health and well being.

Remember that every day presents a fresh opportunity to face life with bravery, resilience, and hope. You may overcome the hurdles offered by RBD and live a meaningful and productive life.

www.ingramcontent.com/pod-product-compliance
Lightning Source LLC
Chambersburg PA
CBHW050827250726

48653CB00006B/2473